THE ELEGANT CRONE

SYDNEY METRICK

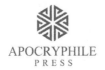

APOCRYPHILE
PRESS

Apocryphile Press
PO Box 255
Hannacroix, NY 12087
www.apocryphilepress.com

Copyright © 2022 by Sydney Metrick
Artwork by Andrea Lozano
Printed in the United States of America
ISBN 978-1-958061-13-8 | paper
ISBN 978-1-958061-14-5 | ePub

Please join our mailing list at
www.apocryphilepress.com/free
We'll keep you uptodate on all our new releases,
and we'll also send you a FREE BOOK. Visit us today!

*I dedicate this book to all the women
who are facing cronehood. May this be a guide.*

CONTENTS

INTRODUCTION

Reflecting on my 74th birthday I realized I was in the midst of a rite of passage. I was about to claim being a crone. This was in 2022. The global COVID-19 pandemic was finally easing up, U.S politics were tumultuous, and a war was raging in Ukraine. It had been a long couple of years, and we were not really sure what was next. As I aged, I found that I, and many of my friends and numerous other women in our 50s, 60s and 70s, were dealing with the issues of our aging bodies—even though our minds are generally intact.

Despite the aging bodies, we have more opportunity than ever to tap into our beauty and power. I find the women friends I have, longstanding and new, are kind, creative, wise, and wonderful. A better bunch of crones would be hard to find. I'd like to share with you a bit about the "Crone" and "croning."

Originally an insult in the male-dominated 14th century, folklore took on the word "crone" in general to signify a grumpy old woman with some sort of supernatural power. As "grumpy old women" have taken a more active role in society, the meaning of "crone" has evolved to indicate an older woman who has lived life and has no use for the judgments of others.

As Jean Shinoda Bolen put it in *Crones Don't Whine: Concentrated Wisdom for Juicy Women*, "A crone is a woman who has found her voice. She knows that silence is consent. This is a quality that makes older women feared. It is not the innocent voice of a child who says, 'the emperor has no clothes,' but the fierce truthfulness of the crone that is the voice of reality. Both the innocent child and the crone are seeing through the illusions, denials, or 'spin' to the truth. But the crone knows about the deception and its consequences, and it angers her. Her fierceness springs from the heart, gives her courage, makes her a force to be reckoned with." The crone lived through childhood, puberty, and fertility to step into the new role of wise woman.

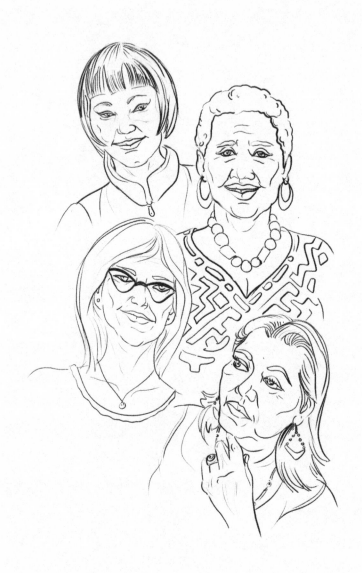

ENTERING CRONEHOOD

Beautiful young people are accidents of nature,
but beautiful old people are works of art.
—*Eleanor Roosevelt*

In the twelve archetypes described by psychiatrist Carl Jung, the crone represents the wise woman. Jung's idea of the collective unconscious, the shared themes and memories of all humanity, describes energies we all carry within that underlie thoughts and behaviors. As women in our 50s, 60s, 70s, and later, we can step away from the "shoulds" and "musts" of society and look at what has formed us throughout those years. This is important for us to truly become wise elders.

By the time we enter the world of the crone the fabric of who we are is woven by the threads of the many relationships we've had—personal and professional; superficial and deep; difficult and easy.

The basis of croning is...determining who we are at the core, how all our life experiences have melded into a firm identity. Accepting that is the basis of croning.

Becoming a crone, claiming your wisdom, may or may not be an easy process. It often takes a particular effort. I've found one means of doing this is by creating a gratitude journal. I began my journal using the wheel of life I employ when coaching. The wheel is a tool that helps break down the relationships you have with the various expressions of your life. It is also a tool that helps you determine your current level of satisfaction and shows you where you might wish to make changes by setting goals.

My wheel categorizes my relationships into ten areas: friends, family, health, home, career, finances, creative expression, community, personal growth, and (life partner?) significant other. These relationships have formed the basis of my gratitude journal. The journal led to a life review.

Looking at your life and seeing what there is to be grateful for is not a difficult task. However, using all or some of the above-named categories and going back through the years of your life is likely to be an intricate process. For example, as you go back and review your relationships with the friends you've had over the decades, you think about friends who have passed through your life, those who've remained, and those who have passed away. In contemplating those relationships, become aware of what each relationship meant to you and how being in that relationship influenced the person that you are now.

Revisiting relationships with friends leads to going over relationships with parents, teachers, bosses, colleagues, neighbors, and others who may have had an impact on your development. Everyone we encounter leaves a mark. How are you marked? How have you marked others?

The same type of review holds true in each of the other categories. Think about the relationship you've had with homes. The homes you lived in, the locations, how much space you had, what your life was like in each home—all have influenced the person you currently are.

Doing a life review is like reading the story of your life.

When you arrive at the present you have a well-developed sense of who you've been and who you've become, so you are prepared to write the next chapter. You looked at all the people and things that contributed to who you currently are—the heroine of your story. In understanding the complexity of your life experiences, you can begin to appreciate what it means to be a crone, or wise woman.

Think of the ancient symbol of the ouroboros—the snake eating its tail. It represents the constant process of transitioning into a new experience of reality. That new reality is your next chapter.

You have decades of experiences that have contributed to your knowledge and strength. It's up to you to acknowledge and claim that strength. I am reminded of the quote on the cover of *Notebook for Christians and Priests*: "The devil whispered in my ear 'you're not strong enough to withstand the storm.' Today I whispered in the devil's ear, 'I am the storm.'"

Rite of Passage

Separation

Transition

Incorporation

THE RITE OF PASSAGE

"I'm baffled that anyone might not think women get more beautiful as they get older. Confidence comes with age and looking beautiful comes from the confidence someone has in themselves." —Kate Winslet

Becoming a crone doesn't just happen. Aging does happen. In *The Velveteen Rabbit*, Margery Williams describes the difference:

"You become. It takes a long time. That's why it doesn't happen often to people who break easily, or have sharp edges, or who have to be carefully kept. Generally, by the time you are Real, most of your hair has been loved off, and your eyes drop out and you get loose in your joints and very shabby.

"But these things don't matter at all, because once you are Real you can't be ugly, except to people who don't understand."

Claiming cronehood means undertaking a rite of passage. We have numerous rites of passage throughout our lives, and when honored with ceremony these transitions have greater meaning. For example, think of getting married in court versus having a wedding with family, friends, special clothing, food, words, and photos to provide memories.

A rite of passage has three parts. Leaving behind that which previously identified you (the separation phase), transition (here you find what is known as the threshold rites), and incorporation (claiming the new identity). Having a ritual or ceremony, with reflection or by participating in a crone circle, can make the transition to cronehood easier.

Rite of Passage

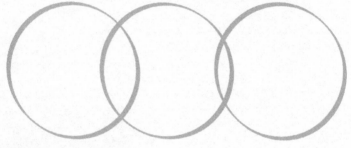

Separation

SEPARATION

The separation phase typically begins as you experience senescence—when you find you look older, need bodily repairs or replacements, experience the loss of friends or family members, or have children leaving home or marrying and having their own children. As these things occur you start seeing yourself differently. The look, the abilities, and the role that had identified you change. This difference may be startling and sometimes difficult to accept. At this time, you're moving away from an earlier stage in life, just as you moved from childhood to adolescence and from adolescence to adulthood. For many, this stage means dealing with grief. The past remains behind you, and you may experience a sense of loss.

In the transition stage you can address the pain of various losses and look at the gifts that remain.

Rite of Passage

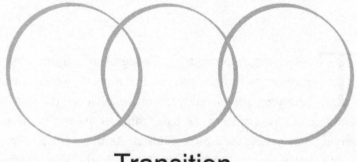

Transition

TRANSITION

The life review is one way to address the transition stage. In this, the waning stage of your life, you look at what you keep and what you release. Lessons learned are part of your identity. However, keeping *how you learned the lessons* is optional. It can be painful saying goodbye to people and things that had once been important. It's important to acknowledge the pain. It may or may not lessen over time depending on how you deal with pain, what support systems you have, and what else is going on in your life.

Your transition may be brief, but it's more likely that processing decades of memories and experiences and coming to a new sense of self will take a while. Even once you have negotiated this stage, it's likely it will not be completed for some time.

As you get older you will understand more and more that it's not about what you look like or what you own, it's all about the person you've become. (*Anonymous*)

I am a "baby boomer." The boomers, born between 1946 and 1964, represented approximately one-fifth of the population of the United States according to 2019 figures. We are the longest-lived generation in history—although, that's not likely to stand given medical advances. We lived through the Cuban Missile Crisis, the civil rights movement, and the Vietnam War, as well as the summer of love, Beatlemania, and the moon landing. And we are becoming crones in a time of turmoil. Independence is a hallmark of our lives as the world rapidly changes. Our independence requires a transformation on a personal level.

Marion Woodman, author, poet, analytical psychologist, and women's movement figure, wrote this in her autobiographical book, *Bone: Dying into Life:*

> What does it mean to be an elder in this culture? What are my new responsibilities? What has to be let go to make room for the transformations of energy that are ready to pour through the body-soul? I don't want to be here if I can't carry my own weight. As life asks new things of me, I feel I must pause, go inward, and ask, "What is my weight now? What are my new values? Who am I and not-I at this stage? Do I have the courage to live with this evolving me?
>
> Negotiating this phase is especially important as you run up against cultural beliefs and values. With ageism rampant in our society, part of your strength in claiming the inner crone is avoiding the trap of external pressures. As Julia Cameron once said, "As with all things, there is a time of dormancy, a time of germination, a time of fruition and harvest. We must be patient with these things in our heart. We must develop patience and an open mind—a very open mind." [1]

Once inspired to claim your cronehood, you may wish to create a ceremony of celebration as part of the process. Doing your own ceremony can be very meaningful. If you've done a life review, you might find a way to transform your thoughts and writings into an ongoing reminder. A journal is one form of remembrance; an altar, another.

A ritual with a group of women undergoing a similar transition can be especially powerful. Having a ceremony where you've invited friends to celebrate with you and documenting the event is yet another possibility.

I participated in a croning ritual for a friend on her 70th birthday. Each of her long-time friends brought a gift that symbolized the value of the woman and the relationship we each had with her over the years. One woman brought a small crystal ball to symbolize clarity and knowledge. Another brought a photo book that highlighted many past events. A childhood friend brought a recipe for a kind of cookie they used to eat after school each day. A gilded mirror symbolized her beauty, and a set of stacking matryoshka dolls represented the children she'd nurtured.

While this was a one-time ceremony, another option for finding how to incorporate the wisdom you hold is to become part of a crone circle. Here is an idea from the Crones Council: "[There is something] called a spiritually based group which focuses on honoring elder women together to create a nurturing, mutually supportive, and confidential environment in which to express and explore their experiences of aging and the sacred passing of time. This type of group provides each woman a place to speak, a place for her story to be told and acknowledged. In addition, crone circles intend to recognize, celebrate, and encourage members in all aspects of the feminine archetype by encouraging qualities such as these: creativity, vitality, spiritual life, joy, service to others, recognition of individuality, and power of being an elder woman coming into her own."[2]

Ego psychologist Erik Erikson characterized eight stages of psychosocial development. The final stage, beginning at approximately age 65, is *Integrity vs. Despair*. In this stage you look back at your life and come away with either a sense of fulfillment or one of regret. Fulfillment includes self-acceptance, wholeness, and wisdom. While we all have times in our past that can arouse regret, fulfillment also includes acknowledging those incidents, moving on, and being OK with where and who you are now.

As you negotiate the transition stage you are redesigning your life. In doing so you're primarily working not only with memories but also with creative imagination. One of my favorite quotes on the topic is by Paul Meyer: "Whatever you vividly imagine, ardently desire, sincerely believe and enthusiastically act upon...must inevitably come to pass!"

Rite of Passage

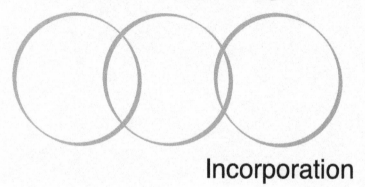

Incorporation

INCORPORATION

As you participate in these practices you will want to incorporate your experiences into your life. You get to claim being a crone and all that goes with it. That does not mean you'd be ever free from self-defeating thoughts or society's influence. It does mean that you have adopted a new, more confident, and self- accepting identity. As Harvey Specter in the television show *Suits* said, "Ever loved someone so much you would do anything for them? Well, name that someone yourself and do whatever the hell you want."

Self-acceptance is a slippery concept. The implication is that you give up comparisons. You do not compare your current self to a younger self unless it's to acknowledge growth. You do not compare yourself to others—that leads to unhappiness.

So, let's say you've been working on the three phases of a rite of passage and you have no difficulty claiming yourself as a crone. What will be different in your life? I like to think it will be full of being a badass: not at all ladylike, pushing boundaries, speaking my mind, and generally doing what I want.

Since aging women have few models of positive aging in society and in the media, it's important to embody independence while gaining visibility and validation. Unlike in years past, each of you must hold fast to the positive aspects of the crone.

> The original Crones of the matriarchal community were women past the age of menopause, in whom the blood of life no longer appeared outside the body. Rather than the cessation of menstruation being a sign of a complete disappearance, the assumption was that the retained blood was the source of wisdom in aged mothers—just as in the stage of fertility that blood had supported the creation of new life. Thus, once menopause was complete, the woman became a Crone, or a Grandmother, with a meaning considerably different from the one we generally know today. The term "Grandmother" meant a "grand" Mother-image and "Mother" meant the goddess of all —life, death, and birth. It was the job of all Crones to assist people in dying or welcome souls in through the birthing ceremonies.[1]

As you can see, the image of the crone has been and can continue to be one of great power. In the New International Version of Proverbs, verse 3:15 says, "She is more precious than rubies; nothing you desire can compare with her." In the New Living Translation, the line is "Wisdom is more precious than rubies; nothing you desire can compare with her." Both describe the crone.

Think of your Self as a multi-faceted jewel with each facet reflecting various aspects of your beauty and wisdom.

"The developmental task of the Crone Stage is sharing wisdom. In Neolithic times, Crone women were the tribal matriarchs. Their heightened awareness of human nature yielded great insight and they were the source of wise counsel for important decisions. Spiritually, this is the Mastery phase. The

Wise Woman teaches knowledge gained from her skills and life experience."[2]

While you may not see yourself literally as a teacher, you are constantly teaching by the ways you interact with the world and with others. In your transition you've likely become more thoughtful. You can hold being thoughtful as an intention. You can decide which parts of your story have given you meaning and would be valuable to hold and to share.

The archetype of the wise woman is universal. "The Wise Woman, also called the Wise Crone, is one of narrative's oldest, most enduring archetypes. In the Wise Woman, compassion and kindness intersect with magic, mystery, and nature. She is, in a sense, the Spiritual in human form."[3]

Western culture has several wise women. Think of Glinda, the older and kinder good witch in the Oz tale, Frances McDormand in *Nomadland*, and older, independent, and intrepid woman. We even have a few real-life wise women, including Ruth Bader Ginsberg with her brilliance and fair-mindedness, Jane Goodall and her dedication, or the magnificently creative Alice Walker.

Across cultures older women often free themselves from their societal constraints. It is a common enough occurrence that Anthropologist Margaret Mead noted that, "There is no greater power in the world than the zest of a post-menopausal woman."

There are many remarkable older women. Tao Porchon-Lynch is a 93-year-old yoga teacher who can still support her whole body on her hands.

Sister Madonna Buder is known in the fitness community as the "Iron Nun." Though in her 80s, she has completed more than *325 triathlons,* including 45 Ironman distances.

Older women have skills and interests ranging from athletes to actors, artists to activists, from teachers to tech writers, counselors to chefs, and more.

As you claim your identity as a crone, you let go of stories you have about what defines you, the way you think about yourself. It's important to ignore the voices that say, "You can't" or "You're not." Taking a stand for self-acceptance might be a bit wobbly. But consider this conversation between Alice (in Wonderland) and the Red Queen: "There's no use trying," said Alice; "one can't believe in impossible things." "I daresay you haven't had much practice," said the Queen. "When I was your age, I always did it for half an hour a day. Why, sometimes I've believed as many as six impossible things before breakfast." (*Lewis Carroll*)

It need not be impossible or even difficult to claim being a crone. We all age and there is no fountain of youth. Even if there was, would you really want to return to the age of 30 again? At the *Radically Reframing Aging* event in 2022, Actress Jamie Lee Curtis is reported to have said, "This word 'anti-aging' has to be struck. I am pro-aging. I want to age with intelligence and grace, and dignity and verve, and energy."[4]

As an actress she can adapt to many different roles. It is just as possible to be old as young, kind as manipulative, lovely as plain. As you take a stand for being a crone, step into your best expression of what a crone can be. Feeling different in an older body and looking different in the mirror can cause that internal saboteur to tell you you've lost value along with your youth. Finding ways to love the body and the face you have at each age —even seeking images and stories of older women you can use as models for loving yourself—are ways to begin to appreciate and express yourself as a crone. As the oft quoted Rabbi Hillel said, "If I am not for myself, who will be for me? If I am only for myself, what am I? And if not now, when?"

Self-expression is an interesting concept to contemplate. I was reading a study on the impact of the creative arts on indigenous societies. Self-expression through the arts can be healing to the individual physically, emotionally, mentally, and spiritually. Being a crone means declaring with confidence that you are an elder—a holder of wisdom. It is unfortunate that the word elderly generally puts in mind frailty. The difference in the words is important. In some traditions, the crone is the eldest version of the triple goddess. The maiden is associated with the waxing moon, the promise of new beginnings and coming into womanhood. The mother, or full moon, represents nurturing, caring protection, ripeness, and fertility. The crone is the waning moon, related to wisdom, death, and recreation.

Elderhood occurs in the second half of life. According to Swiss psychiatrist Carl Jung, there are seven tasks we must negotiate:

- Task One: Face the certainty of death.
- Task Two: Review, reflect upon, and sum up your life.
- Task Three: Let go of roads not taken.
- Task Four: Let go of the dominance of the ego.
- Task Five: Encounter and honor the Self.
- Task Six: Articulate our own *raison d'être*.
- Task Seven: Engage creativity.

LEAVE YOUR MARK

An older woman was asked by a child if she were young or old. "My dear," she replied, "I have been young a very long time."

When reading *Carved in Bone* a specific line stuck with me. The protagonist, anthropologist Dr. Bill Brockton, says, "I've had students tell me years after they've graduated and went out to work for medical examiners or police departments or museums, that I had a big influence on their career path. I think we all leave an imprint on the world, and on the people we cross paths with, sometimes in ways we don't fully understand."[5]

Everyone leaves a mark on the world and the people around them. As a crone, you have the ability to examine the marks you have left—good, bad, or indifferent—and shape the marks you have yet to make.

The book, *Wise Women: A Celebration of Their Insights, Courage, and Beauty*, by Joyce Tenneson, features 85 photographs of women whose ages range from 65 to 100. Each of these women, some celebrities, some not, shared "what it means to them to have lived and grown in strength as a woman during the course of their long lives." These crones have done Jung's tasks five, six, and seven; they have made their mark and are continuing to do so—despite society's attempts to shove them in a dark corner.

For some women, Croning Ceremonies serve as an ideal way to make a statement about that passage. 'I see so many people fighting the aging process,' says Sandra Bury, another Des Moines-area woman who went through the [Croning] Ritual. 'I wanted to celebrate that to become old is a gift. I didn't want to be afraid of it.'[6]

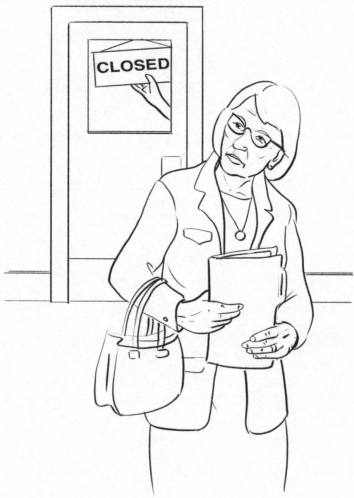

THE IMPACT OF THE FOCUS
ON YOUTH—AGEISM

Some people try to turn back their odometers. Not me, I want people to know "why" I look this way. I've travelled a long way and some of the roads weren't paved. —Will Rogers

D r. Robert N. Butler coined the term *ageism* in 1969. As the founding Director of the National Institute on Ageing as well as the Founder, Chief Executive Officer, and President of the International Longevity Center, you could say that Dr. Butler was the father of modern Gerontology. He defined ageism as "a process of systematic stereotyping of and discrimination against people because they are old...." In his later writings, Butler referred to aging as "the neglected stepchild of the human life cycle."

In a culture that is as youth-oriented as ours, ageism is so ingrained it is an invisible prejudice—especially against women. Think about Marilyn Monroe in the 1953 classic *Gentlemen Prefer Blondes*. Her classic rendition of "Diamonds Are a Girl's Best Friend" includes the line, "men grow cold as girls grow old." Popular culture has been shoveling the concept for decades.

In January 2022, the Columbine Health Systems Center for

Healthy Aging noted that there are nearly 47 million adults over the age of 65 in the United States. Further, "80 percent of adults over the age of 50 have experienced age-based discrimination during their day-to-day."[1]

After that enticing introduction, the article went on to cite a study "aimed to understand younger people's views on aging throughout the world." The study involved questioning over 3,000 college students from 26 cultures in six different continents.

The result? "Across all cultures, there was a consensus that aging comes with a decrease in physical attractiveness, everyday tasks, and learning new things. At the same time, cultures agreed that aging comes with an increase in general knowledge, wisdom, and respect."

Basically, according to college students, getting old means you can do less, but you're smarter and get more respect.

The World Values Survey (WVS), which is an ongoing research project conducted by social scientists around the globe, does not agree.

After analysis of data gathered from over 83,000 people of all age groups in 57 countries about their feelings on aging, the World Health Organization (WHO) noted that 60 percent of survey respondents "reported that older people are not respected." Additionally, "[t]he lowest levels of respect were reported in high income countries."[2]

More recently, the WHO reported that "ageism has serious and wide-ranging consequences for people's health and well-being. Among older people, ageism is associated with poorer physical and mental health, increased social isolation and loneliness, greater financial insecurity, decreased quality of life and premature death. An estimated 6.3 million cases of depression globally are estimated to be attributable to ageism."[3]

Since childhood, society has been training women to project a particular image. It starts with little girls in pink dresses with "good hair" and moves on to the preteen peer pressures, the need to be thin enough, and the desire to impress boys. Magazines for girls and women are full of articles of how we "should be" and what we "should do." We see models with bodies only a small percentage of girls and women actually have. Anorexia and bulimia are common in girls and women.

In 2021 CNBC had an article reporting that the diet and weight loss business is a $71 billion industry, with 45 million people going on a weight-loss program each year in the U.S. alone. The negative social stereotypes persist through the decades. In addition to the weight gain that accompanies many of us as we age, we also find sagging body parts, drier skin, possibly age spots, and certainly wrinkles. We are likely to wonder if we are less attractive than we previously were.

Rather than lamenting the changes, the ceremonies of a rite of passage, especially when done with others, can help us to accept the bodies we live in as our bodies—the home we have lived in all our lives, which have carried us through all the many experiences we've had.

Because in a culture where older women become invisible, we succumb to the promises of the beauty industry. We have no preparation for the transition to being elders. I recall asking one of my aunts who entered her ninth decade, "why didn't anyone tell me what aging would be like?"

There is hope. There are amazing women that have aged in the public eye. The combination of their age and continuing beauty act as a continuous challenge to everyday ageism.

Brooke Shields is one such woman. At 57 years of age, the actress, model, and entrepreneur talked about ageism and her work with Clos du Bois's "Long Live" campaign. "'What they were trying to do was flip the script on ageism,' says Shields. 'There's this misconception—like calling Chardonnay an 'old person's wine' and putting it aside—but truth be told, like wine, we get better with age.'" She went on to add, "it's about changing the narrative to talk about vitality and confidence. You hit this certain age and there's a richness to you. You're just beginning new things."[4]

Another challenge to agism is Betty White. Her film and television career spanned more than 70 years and she established herself as a force in front of, behind, and off camera. In 2012, when speaking to reporters about casting for *The Lorax*, producer Chris Meledandri said, "Betty White is...this phenomenon with Betty White is so wonderfully amazing, it's like in a world where ageism runs rampant, out of left field suddenly the country decides to celebrate Betty White and she becomes cool at 90. It's remarkable."[5]

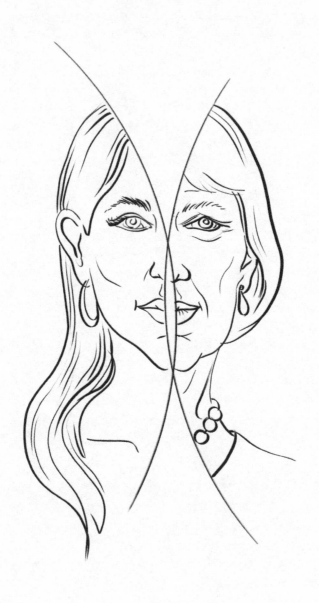

COSMETIC ENHANCEMENT

Native American cultures have a deep respect for the acceptance of our human imperfection. When weaving a rug, they will purposely include a flaw. This serves as a reminder that, while all that is humanly made is imperfect, it yet can reflect the beauty, reverence, care, and love of true creation. —Diane Berke in The Gentle Smile: Practicing Oneness in Daily Life

Respect for the aged is missing in our ageist society—a society in which, for many, looking old is worse than being old and they take steps to shift the balance.

In her book *Elderhood*, Louise Aronson says "An internet search of the term *anti-aging* yields over forty-six million hits. The first of many items that come up are tips, secrets and routines...beauty product, and clinics that promise to help minimize the impact of aging on skin, body and mind. The most frequently used words include *prevent, reversing*, and *corrective*, followed by *age spots, hormones* and *wrinkles...*"[1]

The website of a "facelift specialist" advertises: a more natural younger you; minimize age and maximize beauty.

I spoke with a number of women who underwent facial enhancements.

A 69-year-old woman from New York told me she had her upper and lower eyelids fixed as people told her she looked tired. As an artist she didn't like how she saw herself aesthetically and wanted to be more attractive. She went ahead to have a facelift, nose job, chin implant, and liposuction on her stomach and thighs. She describes herself as "very pro cosmetic surgery."

Another woman, only one year older, related an anecdote about traveling with her daughter who kept telling her she looked angry. One day she looked in the mirror and thought, "Oh my god, I do look angry." Having come from a family in which there was a lot of pressure to look good, and being a performer, she decided to undergo an SMAS facelift and brow lift. The SMAS procedure lifts sagging skin, repositions fat pads in the cheeks, tightens the underlying muscle of the neck and mid- to lower-face, and removes excess skin. She says it was a long recovery and she wishes it was more like how she pictured what she wanted. "I still look like me, but it took me a long time to get used to it."

Personally, I prefer how D. H. Lawrence defined beauty:

"Beauty is an experience, nothing else. It is not a fixed pattern or an arrangement of features. It is something felt, a glow or a communicated sense of fineness."[2]

I talked with a 73-year-old friend, who had microblading done on the recommendation of one of her friends. The goal was to achieve a more youthful look. She said it didn't have the desired effect, was extraordinarily painful, and she'd never do it again. She'd also had filler put into her upper lip to rid herself of the lines common to smokers. She was pleased with this procedure, and commented she thought she looked healthier. (That she quit smoking probably also helped.)

One woman asked, why look a way that doesn't make you feel good? Her series of plastic surgeries and facial enhancements began in her 40s when she was in the fashion industry and looking good was mandatory. Now she considers getting work done simply as maintenance. At the age of 77, she looks damn good.

I interviewed aesthetician Lizzie Malave who worked for a cosmetic dermatologist. Living in the Chicago area she said most clients were affluent white women. Clients typically said they weren't happy with their appearance; they felt they didn't look like themselves anymore. They'd sign up for Botox, filler, chemical peels, or microdermabrasion—sometimes several things at once. And this became a regimented routine for many women. The doctor only occasionally told a patient they'd had enough.

Lizzie said she felt for some women, it was a confidence boost, but there were others who seemed they just weren't happy with themselves and hoped cosmetic procedures would fix things.

Alan Rickman's film, *The Winter Guest*, gives us a glimpse into that unhappiness when the mother, Elspeth (Phillida Law), is looking in the mirror and speaking to her daughter Frances (Emma Thompson):

Elspeth: What do I look like?
Frances: Fine.
Elspeth: Is that my face?
Frances: You look great.
Elspeth: You should change on the inside. I get a fright looking in the mirror. I'm the same inside as I was at 17. I hate my old face.

I don't know if a procedure would have made her feel better.

To give the Devil his due, not all cosmetic procedures require surgery and are minimally invasive. And in an environment concerned with looks, people entering the dating scene or changing jobs frequently feel the need to look younger. The numbers agree.

The American Society of Plastic Surgeons reported Americans over 55 underwent almost 50,000 more cosmetic procedures in 2018 than in 2017. Roughly 4.2 million procedures took place in 2018; of those procedures, two-thirds of all face-lifts and roughly half of all eyelid surgeries, forehead lifts, and lip augmentations were for people 55 and older.[3]

One clinic's FAQ states:

"Cosmetic surgery is very common. Every year, providers do more than 15 million cosmetic surgery procedures in the United States. More than 13 million of those are minimally invasive procedures.

"...These procedures are more common among adults between 40 and 54. Women get around 92% of cosmetic surgery procedures."[4]

These statistics apply not only to Caucasian women. "Non-Caucasian patients presenting for cosmetic surgery tend to have similar motivations and desires as those of their Caucasian counterparts."[5]

Dra. Daniela Bañuelos is a dermatologist in the Lake Chapala area of Jalisco, Mexico. Because she works for a medical center where the doctors must speak English, the majority of her patients are from the U.S. and Canada, though about 20-30% are Mexican. She tells me that even if people come to her office for other reasons, they typically will ask about cosmetic treatments towards the end of the visit. The number one request is for a whole skin care routine. Number two is Botox. The third most common request is for filler, and lastly laser or chemical peels.

Patients are likely to return every six months. They say that when they look better, they feel better. Since they are not prepared for the visual effects of aging, they find it hard to accept. Facial treatments help.

When you can't look good in person, you can look good on paper, with the help of photoshop and other tools,. However, reality is bound to enter at some point.

Kate Winslet revealed she sent the promotional poster for HBO's *Mare of Easttown* back twice, demanding removal of the heavy photoshopping on her face. "They were like, 'Kate, really, you can't,' and I'm like, 'Guys, I know how many lines I have by the sides of my eye, please put them all back.'"[6]

As Naomi Wolf put it in her book *The Beauty Myth*, "To airbrush age [off] a woman's face is to erase women's identity, power, and history... We as women are trained to see ourselves as cheap imitations of fashion photographs, rather than seeing fashion photographs as cheap imitations of women."

Women undergo surgeries and procedures to "look more like our idea of how we should look" — but also, in many cases to please possible mates. It's not just facial enhancements that are popular. Changes to one's body and attire are also common. And this is not new — back in 1926 poet Dorothy Parker wrote the phrase, "Men seldom make passes at girls who wear glasses." The additional offense there is that it is not men and women, or boys and girls, but men and girls.

Fashion icon Coco Chanel said, "You can be gorgeous at thirty, charming at forty, and irresistible for the rest of your life." That is the attitude of a crone, and it does not matter what kind of female (woman or girl) a man prefers.

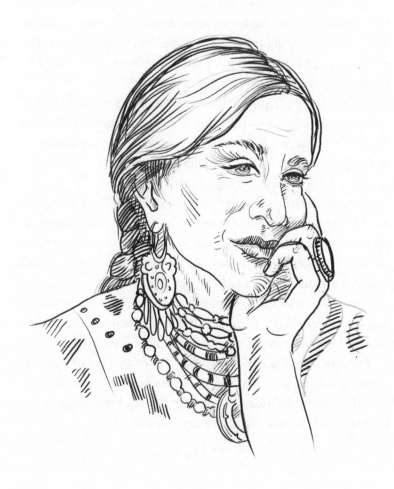

WHAT IS IT LIKE TO BE A CRONE?

Life is not a journey to the grave with the intention of arriving safely in a well-preserved body, but rather to skid in broadside, thoroughly used up, totally worn out, and loudly proclaiming, 'Wow what a ride!'
  – Hunter S. Thompson

Because my experience is not everyone's experience, I took time to interview some of the crones in my life. Here's some of what they had to say.

RENEE HAYES (LONGTIME FRIEND)

Singer songwriter Renee Hayes is a 66-year-old African American woman. When asked how she feels about aging, especially seeing the effects of aging, she replied, "I am not my body." She continued, "I'm more emotionally flexible because things come and go, and I'm less triggered by little things. Also, I'm more relaxed because so many big decisions and life experiences have already happened. Many things have already been decided and I think I've handled them really well.

"I'm more present-oriented and have much more gratitude

about the past and the present. I'm aware that my time is running out and have increased motivation to schedule the things I say I want to do. With creative stuff I'm more of a risk-taker as I realize the stakes are so low. I'm not going to be a star or change the world. I'm relieved that I'm not going to live forever and at some point, I can't worry about things happening in the world, but I do have the opportunity to support the next generation in whatever way that is."

"I believe the second half of one's life is meant to be better than the first half. The first half is finding out how to do it and the second half is enjoying it."—Frances Lear

YOLANDA SAINZ (NEIGHBOR)

Yolanda Sainz is a 65-year-old Mexican woman. She is an interior designer, and a nearly lifelong yoga and meditation teacher. Perhaps because of her spiritual involvement from a young age, she says, "My life is fantastic. I am always happy."

Her guru had taught her that life is a simple adventure and always fantastic.

Her goal now is helping others. She quoted a Spanish phrase, "Quien no vive para server, no sirve para vivir." Who doesn't live to serve, doesn't deserve to live.

Yolanda says many people say life is terrible. "My life is to wake up other people." Yolanda travels to many places in Mexico to teach and help others. Her enthusiasm and vitality are inspiring.

While she looks in the mirror, she says she sees that she is old, but that's not who she is. "I am a young woman in an old body."

ANIN UTIGAARD (COLLEAGUE)

Seventy-one-year-old Caucasian American Anin Utigaard is a licensed MFT, expressive arts therapist, and cancer survivor. Appreciation is a word that came up over and over in our conversation. Anin said she has a new appreciation for her body. She marveled at how well her body responded to treatment with healing. Anin also spoke of the appreciation she has for family and friends, saying they get dearer as we get older. At this stage of life, she knows what she likes and what she doesn't like. She has a huge collection of music and books she continues to enjoy. While she had some of these things in her 30s and 40s, she didn't appreciate them the way she does now.

Her current work involves teaching and mentoring students, which she really enjoys. The increase in confidence she's gained over the years helps her in her work and keeps her going, and she's grateful to know her projects will contribute to what she leaves behind.

"As you get older you will understand more and more that it's not about what you look like or what you own, it's all about the person you've become." (*Anon.*)

Anin has become a person fully living in Erik Erikson's seventh stage of generativity—a sense of contributing to the world.

GENOVEVA CALLOWAY (FRIEND)

Mentoring is a recurring theme in many of women I've spoken with. Genoveva Calloway is a 72-year-old Mexican American woman and past mayor of a California City.

She shared this: "I am feeling proud of being an elder. I have had many experiences that have made me wiser as I grow older and wish to share them with those who want to listen. I currently am a mentor to young women who are in college, and they wish to be involved in their communities, very much like I have been most of my adult life. I currently would like to travel again; read books that I have put off; learn to sew; and begin to write my memoirs for my children, grandchildren, and great-grandchildren.

"What I am struggling with is finding the time to do these things. I have always volunteered in the community, and I am having difficulty 'passing the torch.' I find myself in an 'in-between' space of my past and my future. I have started feeling not wanting to be around groups of my peers because I am afraid of the peer pressure I would perceive as getting to continue staying involved. I am desperately wanting to do less volunteer work and give myself permission to do what I desire to do now. My dear mother passed away this past January. She was 94 years old. I feel that the 'torch' has been passed on to us (my sisters and I, being the three eldest in the family of now 12 siblings).

"I am planning on taking a trip to my mother's hometown in Zacatecas, Mexico with my younger brother, who had taken charge of our mother's care for the past seven years. My mother wanted to go back to her hometown during her last months of life and was not able to do so. I am going to deliver the message to her last few relatives that are still alive, that she thought about them until her last days and wanted to see them. I hope with this trip I too will be able to see and talk to my parents' kin before they pass on to the spirit world. I hope to be able to reflect on my 'in-between' space and return with a clearer mind on implementing and doing the new things I want to do during my last phase of my life. I know that a priority will be to continue mentoring young women in becoming future leaders in the community."

JUNE EGUCHI (NEIGHBOR)

Only one year older than Anin, June Eguchi is a Japanese woman originally from Tokyo. "The biggest gift in my life," reveals June, "at this age is that my hormones and sexual desire have gone away. I no longer need a man in my life. It's all about me. I'm happy every day all the time. Before I thought I wanted a man. I've been married twice, but you have to make compromises in relationships.

"Also, I'm enjoying retirement. I was a medical massage therapist. Now I don't have to be regulated by schedules. Retirement has given me an opportunity to learn who I am. I'm a helper and friendly person.

"I'm comfortable with my body. I'm planning to lose a few pounds I gained during the pandemic, but I don't mind sags and wrinkles. I don't even wear make-up anymore. I'm the most comfortable with me I've ever been.

"In 1972, I had a near death experience. I was in a hepatitis coma for over a week. It led me on a different spiritual path. Our whole life is a lesson."

ANNALEE WEXLER (AUNT)

Annalee Wexler is a 95-year-old Caucasian American great-grandmother. In her early life she was very fortunate to be able to spend many years at home with her husband and children. Now she feels blessed to be in an upscale independent living facility. She has many new friends, and with exposure to a wide variety of people, she's learned to be more open-minded.

Annalee says the last few years have been very good. She's more understanding of people, more accepting. "We're not all alike, we're all different, but different is good, too. You learn from everyone."

DEE GRANT (FRIEND)

Still going strong at 79, Dee Grant is an African American woman who is proud of her excellent health, which she attributes to being active. Participating in the yearly Thrill the World dance as both a dancer and an organizer, taking jazz classes, yoga, and doing lots of walking all help her feel young. She says she now has more time for the arts and needed time for taking care of her husband, who suffers from a series of health issues.

Dee talked about the importance of relationships. Since her daughter married, the two of them have developed a stronger bond, having more similar issues as wives and mothers. Her grandson has been turning to her for advice since he's moved out on his own. Friendships, too, have become more meaningful. She has more time to get together and learn about people.

Over the years, Dee developed many skills that have led to her current passion of organizing community events. She said she plans to be even more involved when her husband's care needs lessen.

LETY OLIVEROS (NEIGHBOR)

Lety Oliveros is a 55-year-old Mexican domestic employee. She tells me her life is better in so many ways. She worked long years alone and now has more help, and as a result has more time to spend with her daughters and grandchildren.

Over the years she's gained so much experience that helps her make better decisions and be able to guide her family well. With the help of many of her clients she finally has her own house, which has taken many of her worries away. Surrounded by very good people, she feels her god has put angels in her life.

SYDNEY METRICK

As I said in the beginning of the book, I was 74 in 2021. Having had undiagnosed ADHD until I was in my 50's I never had much confidence. I'd flunked out of college the first time around, but mostly through non-traditional education I managed to earn a doctorate in expressive therapy.

While trying to fulfill the requirement of a master's thesis while I was in school, I struggled for weeks until someone reminded me of the benefit of using an outline. I had the information in my head, and with an outline as a tool I was unstoppable. Since then, I've written or co-written five books, numerous talks, newsletters, and magazine articles.

I now can acknowledge my creative skill as a writer; something I'd never considered in my younger years.

I disproved my earlier lack of self-esteem with my accomplishments and friendships that have continued for as long as 50 years.

I am more confident in every way.

LOLA PICO (NEIGHBOR)

"I love my life because I have many beautiful moments," asserts Lola Pico, a 60-year-old Spanish woman. She says, "When I was young, I was very insecure. Also, I was spontaneous. I didn't think things through. I had an idea and I'd do it."

She's had many jobs, but now she says she's an artist in her life, being creative in many areas. Now Lola says she feels beautiful because she is natural. "I'm about giving service rather than producing." This gives her more power and more security.

She describes herself as very curious. With animation she declares she loves the surprises in life, the discovery. The little things in life give her joy. During the pandemic she began meditating and contemplating more. She says, "When I know more, I know that I know nothing."

LAN SHAW (COLLEAGUE)

57-year-old Lan Shaw is a Chinese American woman who came to the U.S. at age 35. Lan says, "Life is so much fuller in every single aspect. I see so much beauty." She says she had so much ambition as a younger person, having come from a third world country. She was very driven to accomplish her career goals. Now she is a very successful wealth manager.

Lan shared thoughts about her journey. She says her life journey has expanded her horizons. She has so much self-love, so much confidence, and feels so grounded. Her life is whole in many ways. Her son is going to college, she relaunched her life after going through a divorce, and she feels that she's still growing in her life and in her business.

In fact, Lan says she's in the business of changing people's lives. It gives her so much meaning and satisfaction. It feels humbling and an honor to hear her client's stories and be able to help and empower them. She says, "I'm so grateful in my work, my life and my client's life. We're on a journey together. The journey requires me to be humble, to be present."

LEILANI BELL (FRIEND)

For 62 years of her life, Leilani thought she was half Japanese and half white. "My father was from Oklahoma with roots in Ireland, Scotland, and England. My mother was from Japan. When my adult daughter was given a gift of 23andMe to look at her DNA ancestry, she and I realized that there is no Japanese blood whatsoever. Mom admitted she was adopted. Culturally, mom is Japanese, but ethnically, she is Korean."

She now claims 50% Korean blood and is learning about Koreans in Japan to understand her mom's possible story.

Growing up, Leilani only had her paternal grandmother as a role model for "elderly woman." And what an example she was!

"I knew that her boobs sagged and her skin was loose compared to other women I saw. Either she or my parents probably told me it was because of her age. I probably figured it would happen to all women who live long enough."

"I loved her open-mindedness and trusting nature. She never tried to shame me or my sister as my Asian mother did. She gave us just the right amount of freedom.

"I think I may be a lot like my grandmother. I am also a hard worker. I don't bake as much as she does. I like to think of myself as open-minded.... My boobs don't sag to my waist like hers did...."

Not really letting age slow her down, Leilani has found a new role model in her neighbor Marilyn, who's probably 20 years older than Leilani. "I started playing tennis in my 50s thanks to ... Marilyn, who invited me to a tennis clinic at her gym.

"Since starting to play tennis I have met other elderly women who play. They are definitely role models for me now. Connie is 86 and still playing tennis. I think sports like tennis or pickleball keep people young.

"Life is pretty good for me as an elder. I have a beautiful home. In the past I have bemoaned being single, but it is not a bad life. I have friends of both genders, straight and gay, and a decent support group. I work as a school nurse, earning a decent living, and I look forward to retirement very soon.

"Pros of being older and still employed include financial stability, ability to own nice things and choose one's own destiny to some extent. Cons of being older include changes in skin appearance, including getting more wrinkles on the skin, the belly wanting to bulge more, difficulty losing weight. I think that occasional difficulty sleeping came with age for me.

"I think some things *tend to go with aging,* like wisdom and maturity—*but not necessarily.* A male friend of mine a couple of years older than me comes to mind as an immature 65-year-old. I like to think that I have matured and become wiser through learning and increased self-awareness." Leilani sums up her healthy aging well with the saying "Progress, not perfection."

THE LONG AND SHORT OF
BEING A CRONE

Don't prioritize your looks, my friend,
they won't last the journey.
Your sense of humor though, will only get better.
Your intuition will grow and expand like a majestic cloak of
*   wisdom.*
Your ability to choose your battle will be fine-tuned to perfection.
Your capacity for stillness, for living in the moment, will blossom.
And your desire to live each and every moment will transcend all
*   other wants.*
Your instinct for knowing what (and who) is worth your time,
*   will grow and flourish like ivy on a castle wall.*
Don't prioritize your looks, my friend,
they will change forevermore,
that pursuit is one of much sadness and disappointment.
Prioritize the uniqueness that makes you you, and the invisible
*   magnet that draws in other like-minded souls to dance in your*
*   orbit.*
These are the things which will only get better.
—Donna Ashworth, from 'To The Women'

In short, we all have found value in our older years.

I happened to run across this post on Facebook[1] and was surprised by how fitting it is:

What does it feel like to be old?

The other day, a young person asked me:—What did it feel like to be old?

I was very surprised by the question, since he did not consider me old. When he saw my reaction, he was immediately embarrassed, but I explained that it was an interesting question. And after reflection, I concluded that getting old is a gift.

Sometimes I am surprised at the person who lives in my mirror. But I don't worry about those things for long. I wouldn't trade everything I have for a few less gray hairs and a flat stomach. I don't scold myself for not making the bed, or for eating a few extra "little things." I am within my rights to be a little messy, to be extravagant, and to spend hours staring at my flowers.

I have seen some dear friends leave this world before they had enjoyed the freedom that comes with growing old.

– Who cares if I choose to read or play on the computer until 4 in the morning and then sleep until who knows what time?

I will dance with me to the rhythm of the 50s and 60s. And if later I want to cry for some lost love...I will!

I'll walk down the beach in a swimsuit that stretches over my plump body and dive into the waves letting myself go, despite the pitying looks of the bikini-wearers. They'll get old too—if they're lucky...

It is true that through the years my heart has ached for the loss of a loved one, for the pain of a child, or for seeing a pet die. But it is suffering that gives us strength and makes us grow. An unbroken heart is sterile and will never know the happiness of being imperfect. I am proud to have lived long enough for my hair to turn gray and to retain the smile of my youth, before the deep furrows appeared on my face.

Now, to answer the question honestly, I can say:—I like being old, because old age makes me wiser, freer!

I know I'm not going to live forever, but while I'm here, I'm going to live by my own laws, those of my heart. I'm not going to regret what wasn't, nor worry about what will be. The time that remains, I will simply love life as I did until today, the rest I leave to God.

Lunyta—in Oldsmar, Florida.

When used as a model, these words can make the transition into cronehood easier.

Not everyone can live without regrets and experience depression with aging.

Some women find, despite the confidence and wisdom that may come with aging, there can be a downside. For those who raised families and are no longer involved, or women who had careers that served as a large part of their identity, depression might dilute the ability to enjoy cronehood.

You may feel a lack of purpose, experience sleep issues, or lethargy. You may have lost intellectual stimulation, daily structure, or important relationships. Your home situation may have changed if you live with a spouse. The fears that come with aging bodies and the loss of others in your age group can have a negative impact that is difficult to overcome.

Fears around ageing are real and reasonable. That is why finding supportive and nurturing involvements can make a big difference. A crone circle is a way to participate in life and find meaning. Remember, you always have the capacity to transform fears into trust, confidence, and contentment.

The symbolism of a circle is of transformation and wholeness. Being part of a circle enables change to occur on many levels. A crone circle can provide the support you need to find the wise elder within that is not only acceptable, but magnificent.

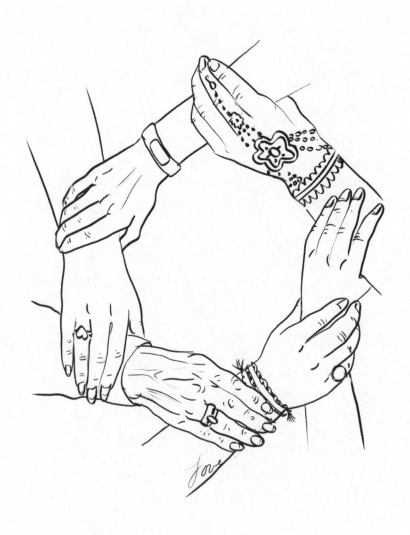

CREATING A CRONE CIRCLE

"I've got silver in my hair,
   Gold in my heart,
   And steel in my veins,
   …and I know my worth"

Women's circles have existed for thousands of years. The earliest circles may have been around new or full moons, cooking fires, child feeding. Circles also focused on ritual, storytelling, cleansing, healing, and various types of support.

"Back in the 80s a feminist movement began with the idea that meeting in circle was a feminine way to share stories and promote healthier communication. It was taking place with Western women and also as far away as Africa. They were remembering, consciously or unconsciously, the importance of circle and healthier ways of gathering."[1]

"In the circle a space was created for connection, enriching peer-to-peer communication or healing, and bonds were strengthened."[2]

When you are ready to claim being a crone, being part of a circle with other women sharing similar experiences can be very valuable. To create a croning circle you'd follow the five steps of the ritual process.

INTENTION

The first stage is intention, in which you determine the purpose of your circle.

What is your need or desire, and what do you feel would be important for others to share? Think about the who, how, when, as well as the why. You may wish to have your circle as a way of bonding with like-minded others and/or a way for people to experience growth and change. Might you want each gathering to have the aspects of a formal ritual or be a more informal and spontaneous group?

PLANNING

In the planning stage you imagine what you want your circle to "look like."

- How many women would you invite and how would you choose them?
- What process would you use to explain the purpose and invite women to the gathering?
- How often would you like to meet?
- What would be a good length for each gathering?
- Where would the gatherings be held? Would the meeting rotate locations?
- Would there be a structure?
- How would you begin and end each meeting?
- Would you want to have an altar?

- Will there be a time for each woman to share and a limit on sharing time?
- How do you imagine achieving support, growth, and change? Is there another purpose, and how do you imagine achieving that?
- What about confidentiality?
- Would the gatherings be open to new participants?
- Might you include activities as well as sharing?
- Would you have food and drink?

PREPARATION

You will want to do some basic preparations for the first meeting. You'll already have invited the women you wish to be part of the circle. Before they arrive, you'll need to prepare the space and have all your notes. As circles are most successful when there is a shared facilitation you can use this first meeting to get input on all the planning points from the women in the group.

Women may have ideas like using a talking stick to make sure each speaker is free from interruptions. Ideas for sharing might include:

- Discussing the energy around the word *crone*.
- What does being a crone mean to you?
- How are you different as an elder?
- What is one thing you learned since the last circle?
- What might be some activities the group may wish to incorporate? (Such as writing thoughts or drawing images that may have come up.)

At this initial gathering the group will decide what they would like future get-togethers to be about. Would bringing a creative activity into each gathering make it more meaningful?

You can consider using clay, paint, music, poetry, sculpture, dance, performance, or whatever appeals to the group.

Perhaps each woman will have tasks to perform in preparation for the first formal circle.

MANIFESTATION

You will likely be the leader of the first formal circle. It's good to thank everyone for participating and share your vision for the circle. This is the time when you carry out everything in the preparation stage. Be prepared for things to be fluid and not evolve exactly as you'd imagined. What's important is that everyone is and feels heard and for the energy to be positive and growth-oriented.

If there is agreement within the group, you may wish to record the session for anyone who may not have been able to attend. Recordings can also be for review of what worked well and what might benefit from change.

In future circles keep in mind that growth is continuous. No matter how far our journey takes us, we will ultimately arrive where we started. Then we will be aware of our true nature.

EVALUATION

You have choices here. You may wish to have each member of the circle share what they think worked or didn't. They may also have new ideas. As it is a group of equals, everyone's thoughts and ideas matter. How will the group carry out their decisions?

According to your original intention, how did it go? Are you satisfied? Is the circle giving you what you had hoped for? Or are you, as the initiator, feeling it's not the right place for you?

The intention behind crone circles is to create a nurturing, supportive, and growth-oriented environment. They can encourage friendships, empowerment, and creativity. Did you succeed in building that type of environment?

Each circle will have its own identity and gatherings may differ from meeting to meeting. It's important that each member feels they are contributing and benefitting from their involvement.

The circles, then, have a sense of fluidity. What was planned may be altered. Certain members may choose to leave, and a leaving process is important. The group may wish to add members at various points. Again, a joining process would be of value.

Some members may develop close friendships and continue to work on issues and growth outside of the circle. They can choose to keep those to themselves or share them with the circle members.

There is no right way. What's right is what works best for all.

CLOSURE OF CIRCLE

After each circle you may want to do a breakdown and break-through evaluation for yourself.

Breakdowns:

- In what ways have you focused on loss?
- What have you given up on?
- What aspects of not accepting being a crone may be holding you back from a good life?
- Where are you settling for less?
- Do you ever say, "I'd be happy if only...?

Breakthroughs:

- In what ways are you being authentic?
- How are you curious about what each day may bring?
- What are some surprises you've enjoyed that have come with aging?
- Have you released attachment to a self-image?
- Are you able to see aging as simply a season, using the time of autumn differently than spring or summer?

Many circles close with a blessing from a chosen culture. I happen to like the Navajo Blessingway Prayer:

In beauty may I walk.
All day may I walk.
Through the returning seasons may I walk.
On the trail marked with pollen may I walk.
With grasshoppers about my feet may I walk.
With dew about my feet may I walk.
With beauty may I walk.
With beauty before me, may I walk.
With beauty behind me, may I walk.
With beauty above me, may I walk.
With beauty below me, may I walk.
With beauty all around me, may I walk.
In old age wandering on a trail of beauty, lively, may I walk.
In old age wandering on a trail of beauty, living again, may I walk.
It is finished in beauty.
It is finished in beauty.

CIRCLES

In researching crone circles, I came across multiple examples with many variations. One group, Hopi Wisdom Teachings, offers several types of groups that meet on-line. These "Wisdom Circles are yearlong and meet monthly. Each Wisdom Circle is completely unique but what emerges and reemerges during the evolution of sitting in a Wisdom Circle is that something ancient, archetypal, and deep is evoked. This magic is not specifically created by the process of the Circle itself, but by the coming together of people for the common and specific purpose of spiritual self-discovery."[3]

Another group in Louisiana holds a grandmother circle. This local group meets in-person and is comprised of women who have lived 50-plus years but are not necessarily grandmothers in the literal sense. "Some of (the women) have been meeting together for many years, and newcomers are welcome…The group is facilitated by a council of four elders who meet bimonthly to arrange for scheduling events. Much is planned to follow the seasonal movements of Mother Earth and the moon cycles. The Grandmothers follow the premise of the Native American Hopi prophecy: 'When the grandmothers speak, the Earth will heal.'"[4]

There is "a deck of cards called *Wisdom of the Crone* (www.wisewomenink.com) that says, 'When you seek the truth, ask a wise woman.' Wise women are all around us and they are calling us to sit at their fire and learn what only wisdom can teach us.

"One of the cards in the crone deck says, 'Sometimes we wonder what legacy we will leave. What song, joke, advice or story will be passed along. Now we can be of great influence. Older women have passion, time, guts, and experience. Some say when the grandmothers speak the Earth will be healed. Look seven generations ahead.'"[5]

The book jacket for *Grandmothers Counsel the World: Women Elders Offer Their Vision for Our Planet* proclaims, "In some Native American societies, tribal leaders consulted a counsel of grandmothers before making any decisions that would affect the whole community."

FULFILLING A NEED

At this time of your life when you could choose to have your life be about something, what would you choose? As Cindy Joseph said, "Aging is just another word for living." You can do or be many things in your crone years. In 1970, Maggie Kuhn formed The Gray Panthers organization in response to her forced retirement from the Presbyterian Church at the age of 65. Those in the organization work towards:

- Creating a humane society—one that puts the needs of people over profits, responsibility over power, and democracy over institutions.
- Eliminating injustice, discrimination, ageism wherever they exist.
- Bringing together young and old, women and men of all backgrounds and orientations, to work in unison, with mutual trust and respect.

According to facts.net, panthers have many qualities which are important in sport, including strength, agility, endurance, ingenuity. The symbolism also connects to grace, protection, beauty, night, magic, inner power, and even the secrets of life and death.

You can see how the symbolism can easily apply to the crone. You are charged with finding your own strength, agility, endurance, ingenuity, grace, and so on. These qualities belong to you and wait for you to fully claim them.

For many women, becoming an elder and claiming strength and beauty is difficult. Some of the things associated with aging are real. We do have more wrinkles, flabby skin, may do things more slowly, or have difficulty remembering things.

That is just the body we live in. That is the body that has taken us on the journey and many adventures.

However, in a survey done by Dr. Barbara Flood[6], 50% of the women surveyed say:

- The experience of aging is better than they expected it would be.
- Older women are no more likely than younger women to report they have a disability. Women 80 and over are significantly more likely to report that they are in good health than are younger women.
- Overwhelmingly they report that their mental health is good.
- Working women are healthier and have a more optimistic reaction to aging and their financial future than their nonworking 'sisters.'
- Women 50 and over feel strongly that many public policy issues are of importance to them, including those that affect improving conditions for all ages of Americans

I used to attend the yearly classic car shows in my area. There were hundreds of restored and cherry cars from the 50s and 60s and even a few from the 30s or 40s. Each car was a work of art. The owners had lovingly replaced or repaired every bit of the cars, and each was stunning.

This is not to suggest you fall into the cosmetic enhancement trap, rather to care for your body as the precious vehicle it is.

As the crone, you are the eldest embodiment of the triple goddess—maiden, mother, crone. As Starhawk describes in the charge of the Star Goddess, let this be your prayer: "Know that your seeking and yearning will avail you not, unless you know the Mystery: for if that which you seek, you find not within yourself, you will never find it without. For behold, I have been with you from the beginning, and I am that which is attained at the end of desire."[7]

AFTERWORD

In writing this book, I learned many things from talking with a wide range of women and doing research. I've found that growing old doesn't have to mean being marginalized, lamenting the loss of youth or beauty, or having few things of importance for a full life.

In the words of Dr. Seuss, "You're only old once." Rather than mourning your younger self, why not look at the gifts aging has given you. It's simply a change of focus and committing to that shift.

I recently called a friend to wish her a happy birthday. In thinking back, we realized we'd been friends for 45 years. I've known her children since they were small, enjoyed every birthday and holiday with them for over 30 years, we have gone through many of life's adventures together. Our friendship is one of the many treasures I've acquired over the years.

"I discovered that age, aging is living. We are born, and we start living, and from the day we're born we start aging. And we continue until the day we die. So aging and living are one in the same."[1]

NOTES

TRANSITION

1. Cameron, Julia. *Faith and Will: Weathering the Storms in our Spiritual Lives* (NY: TarcherPerigree, 2010).
2. Friedrich, Carol and Lehto, Nancy. *How to Start a Crones Circle.* Crones Counsel, 2021. https://tinyurl.com/3wfcneuf, PDF file.

INCORPORATION

1. Ransom, Victoria and Bernstein, Henrietta. *The Crone Oracles: Initiate's Guide to the Ancient Mysteries* (Newburyport: Red Wheel/Weiser, 1994) p. 127
2. Savage, Linda E., PhD. "The Three Stages of a Woman's Life." *The Therapist Directory of San Diego*, 24 Oct. 2016, https://tinyurl.com/yckmvzvj
3. Trippeer, Jordan. "Exploring Female Character Archetypes—The Wise Woman." *Creative Screenwriting*, 7 Jan. 2021, https://tinyurl.com/49kns3f2
4. Beni, Shauna. "Jame Lee Curtis, 63, Says She's 'Pro-Again' And That 'Anti-Aging Has To Be Struck'." *Yahoo! News* 26 March 2022, https://tinyurl.com/f5sa949f
5. Bass, Jefferson. *Carved in Bone.* Kindle ed. Harper, Reissue Edition, 2013.
6. Voss, Melinda. "Guest Post." *DeAnna Lam,* 1 Apr. 2017, https://tinyurl.com/4w5486sa

THE IMPACT OF THE FOCUS ON YOUTH— AGEISM

1. Weintrob, Grace. "Aging Around the World" *Colorado State University*, 28 Jan. 2022, https://tinyurl.com/mu7ea48x
2. "Discrimination and negative attitudes about ageing are bad for your health." *World Health Organization.* 29 Sept. 2016. https://tinyurl.com/yckmkun6
3. "Ageism is a global challenge: UN." *World Health Organization.* 18 March 2021. https://tinyurl.com/njbu4t7h
4. Peters, Terri. "Brooke Shields on how women in their 50s are like wine: 'You hit this certain age and there's a richness to you'" *Yahoo!* 2 May 2022. https://tinyurl.com/378v7rht

5. Radish, Christina. "10 Things to Know About DR. SEUSS' THE LORAX From Our Editing Room Visit; Plus an Interview with Producer Chris Meledandri." *Collider*, 30 Jan. 2012, https://tinyurl.com/ye4njzan

COSMETIC ENHANCEMENT

1. Aronson, Louise. *Elderhood: Redefining Aging, Transforming Medicine, Reimagining Life* (New York: Bloomsbury Publishing Inc., 2019), 87.
2. https://www.azquotes.com/quote/520328?ref=beauty
3. Thompson, Dennis. "More baby boomers opting for cosmetic surgery," *UPI.* 20 June 2019. https://tinyurl.com/fm439v
4. "Cosmetic Surgery & Skincare" *Cleveland Clinic* 21 June 2021. https://tinyurl.com/3nwsf45j
5. Wimalawansa, Sunishka MD, et al. "Socioeconomic Impact of Ethnic Cosmetic Surgery: Trends and Potential Financial Impact the African American, Asian American, Latin American, and Middle Eastern Communities Have on Cosmetic Surgery" *National Library of Medicine*, Aug. 2009, https://tinyurl.com/53thbkte
6. Dowd, Maureen. "Kate Winslet Has No Filter." *The New York Times* 31 May 2021. https://tinyurl.com/4w4defbt

THE LONG AND SHORT OF BEING A CRONE

1. Life's Simple Truths. What does it feel like to be old? Facebook, 22 May 2022, 2:52 pm, https://tinyurl.com/82ncfkh3

CREATING A CRONE CIRCLE

1. Mijares, Sharon Dr. "A Brief History of Circle" *Website of Dr. Sharon Mijares,* 2014. https://tinyurl.com/3vyks63u
2. A.M.A.T.E Center. "Moon Circles: Honoring My Mother" Connecciones, May 2022 p. 26, https://tinyurl.com/46yf38su
3. Grandmother Medicine Song. "Wisdom Teachings" *Hopi Wisdom Teachings,* 16 Feb 2022. hopiwisdomteachings.com/wisdomcircles/
4. "Grandmother Circle." *Women's Center for Healing & Transformation.* 2019. www.womenscenterforhealing.org/grandmother-circle.html
5. Edveeje. "When the Grandmothers Speak." *TreeSisters*, 16 Jan. 2015, https://treesisters.org/blog/when-the-grandmothers-speak
6. Flood, Barbara Dr. "Rewriting the Myth of Women and Ageing" *The Selwyn Foundation.* 24 Sept. 2009. https://tinyurl.com/3d35seuf, PDF file.
7. Starhawk, *The Spiral Dance*, (New York: Harper & Row, Publishers, Inc., 1979) p. 77

AFTERWORD

1. Joseph, Cindy. "Aging is Living." *Boom by Cindy Joseph* 13 Dec. 2016. https://tinyurl.com/bdfh8k78

ACKNOWLEDGMENTS

I'd like to thank all the women who shared their stories with me. I could not have come up with this final product without: my friend and editor, Lorrie Nicoles, who brought it all together; and the wonderful artist, Andrea Lozano.

I gained inspiration from more authors and poets than I could cite, including T.S. Eliot, Caitriona Loughrey, and Suzanne Reynolds. I strongly encourage you to look them up and find some inspiration of your own.

Made in the USA
Monee, IL
30 April 2024

57714917R00049